14 Days Dairy-Free
The Ultimate Dairy-Free and Lactose –Free Meal Plan Cookbook
Breakfast, Lunch, Snack, Dinner and Dessert

By Diana Welkins

*Copyright: Published in the United States by Diana Welkins /
© Diana Welkins
Published 07/14/2015*

All rights reserved. No part of this publication may be reproduced, stored in retrieval system, copied in any form or by any means, electronic, mechanical, photocopying, recording or otherwise transmitted without written permission from the publisher. Please do not participate in or encourage piracy of this material in any way. You must not circulate this book in any format. Diana Welkins does not control or direct users' actions and is not responsible for the information or content shared, harm and/or actions of the book readers.

In accordance with the U.S. Copyright Act of 1976, the scanning, uploading and electronic sharing of any part of this book without the permission of the publisher constitute unlawful piracy and theft of the author's intellectual property. If you would like to use material from the book (other than just simply for reviewing the book), prior permission must be obtained by contacting the author.

Thank you for your support of the author's rights.

Table of Contents

1. Common Food Allergies and How They Affect Your Life

2. Testing For Dairy Allergies

    2.1. Subscribe For Free Updates and New Releases!

3. Day 1

    3.1. Breakfast: Non- Dairy Pancakes

    3.2. Lunch: Crab and Avocado Salad

    3.3. Snack: Bagel Chips

    3.4. Dinner: Jerk Skewers with Black Beans & Rice

    3.5. Dessert: Non-Dairy Chocolate Ice Cream

4. Day 2

    4.1. Breakfast: Turkey Sausage Patties

    4.2. Lunch: Mango Chicken Wraps

    4.3. Snack: Baked Corn Dog Bites

    4.4. Dinner: Pumpkin Curry with Chickpeas

    4.5. Dessert: Dairy-Free Chocolate Chip Cookie Dough Ice Cream

5. Day 3

    5.1. Breakfast: French Toast

    5.2. Lunch: Grilled Hummus and Vegetable Wrap

    5.3. Snack: Crispy Apple Bites

    5.4. Dinner: Lemon Zest Spaghetti with Tuna & Broccoli

  5.5. Dessert: Scrumptious Banana Cookies

6. Day 4

  6.1. Breakfast: Baked Blueberry-Apple Oatmeal

  6.2. Lunch: Chicken Fried Rice

  6.3. Snack: Bean and Chili Dip

  6.4. Dinner: Blackened Tuna Steaks with Mango Salsa

  6.5. Dessert: Ginger Cookies

7. Day 5

  7.1. Breakfast: Almond & Cranberry Granola

  7.2. Lunch:

  7.3. Snack: Curry Potato Wedges

  7.4. Dinner: Sweet and Spicy Chicken

  7.5. Dessert: Apple Enchilada

8. Day 6

  8.1. Breakfast: Toasted Peanut Butter and Banana Sandwich

  8.2. Lunch: Chicken Fajitas

  8.3. Snack: Garlic & Rosemary Bites

  8.4. Dinner: Pineapple Chicken Strips

  8.5. Dessert: Vanilla Vegan Cake

9. Day 7

  9.1. Breakfast: Tropical Breakfast Smoothie

  9.2. Lunch: Turkey Chipotle Chili

  9.3. Snack: Spring Rolls with Ginger Sauce

  9.4. Dinner: Beef & Veggie Beer Chili

  9.5. Dessert: Pineapple Orange Sorbet

10. Day 8

    10.1. Breakfast: Early Sunrise Smoothie

    10.2. Lunch: Smoked Turkey Reuben

    10.3. Snack: Baked Plantain Chips

    10.4. Dinner: Red Whine Beef and Mushroom Sauté

    10.5. Dessert: Homemade Dairy-Free Peach Ice Cream

11. Day 9

    11.1. Breakfast: Banana, Granola, Chocolate Chip Muffins

    11.2. Lunch: Spicy Chicken Pitas

    11.3. Snack: Tossed Edamame with Chile Salt

    11.4. Dinner: Chicken and Squash Casserole

    11.5. Dessert: Fruit Ice Cream

12. Day 10

    12.1. Breakfast: Delightful Danish Puffs

    12.2. Lunch: Ham and Cheese Turnovers

    12.3. Snack: Popcorn Balls

    12.4. Dinner: Carolina-Style Oven-Barbecued Chicken

    12.5. Dessert: Gingersnap Pumpkin Cheesecake

13. Day 11

    13.1. Breakfast: Dairy-Free Scrambled Eggs

    13.2. Lunch: Greek Salad

    13.3. Snack: Caramel Apple Cookies

    13.4. Dinner: Super Quick Cheeseless Pizza

    13.5. Dessert: Orange Delight Cake

14. Day 12

    14.1. Breakfast: Baked Cinnamon Toast

    14.2. Lunch: Horseradish Roast Beef and Vegan Cheddar Cheese Roll-Ups

    14.3. Snack: Peanut Butter-Banana Spirals

    14.4. Dinner: Watermelon Baja Fish Tacos

    14.5. Dessert: Almond Cookies

15. Day 13

    15.1. Breakfast: Gingerbread Pancakes

    15.2. Lunch: Swiss Mushroom and Almond Melt

    15.3. Snack: Tomato Turnovers

    15.4. Dinner: Oriental Beef with Broccoli

    15.5. Dessert: Dairy-Free Brownies

16. Day 14

    16.1. Breakfast: Quinoa Breakfast Bowl

    16.2. Lunch: Chipotle-Lime Grilled Fish Tacos

    16.3. Snack: Pumpkinseed Mix

    16.4. Dinner: Savory Salmon Burgers

    16.5. Dessert: Easy Lemon Bars

17. Meet the Author

18. Additional Recipe Books

19. Sneak Peek

Common Food Allergies and How They Affect Your Life

Food Allergy

A food allergy is whenever a person's immune system, by error, recognizes a protein in the food as hazardous and the immune system will activate an allergic reaction, because it mistakenly perceives that the system is under attack. The scale of allergic reactions to food ranges from mild to extremely severe. Regarding a food allergy, Immunoglobin E (IgE) antibodies are in existence.

Food Intolerance

Food intolerance is an unfavorable reaction or a food hypersensitivity to some kind of food, additive or drink. Discomforts will occur, which can often be delayed, and can occur in one or more internal organs of the body. To a food intolerant individual the allergic reactions can be as agonizing as some food allergy reactions. Each is determined by the individual and the reaction. However in the case of food intolerance, that is non-allergic food hypersensitivity, Immunoglobin E (IgE) antibodies are not present.

Dairy Allergy

A dairy allergy takes place whenever an individual has developed an allergic response to one of the many proteins found in milk, however the most typical culprit is alpha S1-casein. When it comes to a dairy allergy the signs and symptoms may be comparable to lactose intolerance there is however also the possibility of anaphylactic reactions , allergic colitis , gastric distress , skin rashes , hives , atopic dermatitis , a wheeze , oral irritations , headaches , and migraines.

Lactose Intolerance

When it comes to lactose intolerance the entire body is not generating sufficient lactase to be capable of break down the lactose in milk as well as other food or drink products. Several of the symptoms that are considered common are cramps, bloating, flatulence, diarrhea, rumbling tummy and vomiting, particularly in adolescents.

Testing For Dairy Allergies

The best method to check for a dairy allergy would be to eliminate all dairy for 2 weeks , in case you have an allergy you will discover the difference , in some instances right after a couple of days , however some individuals need 10 days to 2 weeks .

Whether it appears that dairy free living will be beneficial to you, then it will help psychologically to learn about these seven advantages of dairy free living.
Throughout the transition time it is beneficial to focus on the fact that living dairy free means:

- Anxiety and stress levels will decrease
- Stamina levels will increase
- Body mass may become healthier (some find they lose unwanted weight is much easier).
- Several tests have confirmed that hyperactivity as well as autism can be improved by dairy free living.
- You should no longer have the feeling of nausea.
- Bodily hormones may become more balanced in some instances, which will help for better moods and overall well being
- Decreased cholesterol and sodium levels in the bloodstream, which is much better for physical health.

Subscribe For Free Updates and New Releases!

I want to thank you for purchasing this book. I hope that this book will be helpful to you and your needs while also helping you maintain and eliminate harmful food allergy complications that can be stressful and destroy your life.

Please take the time to subscribe to my free newsletter for early access to new book releases, free book promotions, and information on how you can keep a healthy digestion with nutritious non-dairy recipes.

Thank you.

Subscribe!

https://tinyletter.com/dwelkins

Additional Recipe Books

Dairy-Free

Envious Cow Non-Dairy Ice Cream: 31 Flavors of Dairy-Free, Paleo, and Vegan Friendly Ice Cream Recipes

Dairy-Free Smoothies: Seriously Yummy Paleo, Vegan, and Gluten-Free Non-Dairy Smoothie

Slice The Dairy: 21 Tasty and Delicious Dairy-Free Pizza Recipes

Vegetarian

Vegetarian Cookout: Scrumptious Barbecue Grilling Recipe Cookbook

Vegetarian Freezer Meal Recipes: Time Saving Vegetarian Freezer Meal Recipes

Vegetarian Lifestyle Cookbook: 20 Delightful Vegetarian Lasagna Recipes

Paleo

30 Days Paleo Diet Breakfast: Ultimate Ready Paleo Diet Breakfast Meal Recipe Cookbook

No Grain, No Gain Sandwich Recipes: Premium Gluten-Free and Paleo Breadless Sandwiches and Wraps Recipes

Author's Page http://www.amazon.com/Diana-Welkins/e/B00WS76QHY/ref=ntt_dp_epwbk_0

Day 1

3.1. Breakfast: Non- Dairy Pancakes

Yield: 6 Servings

Ingredients

1 cup white flour

3 tablespoons white sugar

2 1/4 teaspoons baking powder

1/4 teaspoon salt

2 1/2 tablespoons dairy-free dairy- free margarine

3/4 cup water

1 eggs or 2 tablespoons water

Instructions

1. Mix the flour, sugar, baking powder, and salt collectively into medium mixing bowl.
2. Melt 2 1/2 Tbsp. of dairy- free margarine in frying pan until well melted.
3. Coat and grease the pan all over.
4. Pour melted dairy- free margarine in a compact bowl then add water and egg (if you want to add egg) and mix well.
5. Combine liquid mixture into the dry ingredients until it is thoroughly moistened.
6. It is fine if the batter becomes lumpy.
7. Prepare the pancakes over medium-high heat on the stove-top (or 375F on electric frying pans).

8. Cook the pancakes until the tops are bubbly and the bottoms have browned.
9. Flip the pancakes over to evenly cook both sides.
10. Serve up warm with dairy- free margarine, honey, brown sugar or maple syrup.

3.2. Lunch: Crab and Avocado Salad

Yield: 4 Servings

Ingredients

Kosher salt

1/2 pound haricots verts or green beans, halved

2/3 cup dairy-free yogurt

3 tablespoons low-fat mayonnaise

1 to 2 tablespoons fresh lemon juice

1/2 cup chopped fresh chives

1/4 cup chopped fresh basil

3 anchovy fillets, chopped

Freshly ground pepper

1/2 pound lump or claw crabmeat

1 Hass avocado, halved, pitted and diced

3 romaine hearts, chopped

1 1/2 cups whole-wheat croutons

1 pint cherry tomatoes, halved

Instructions

1. Produce a small pan of salted water to a boil.
2. Add in the haricots verts and cook until crisp-tender for approximately 3 to 5 minutes.
3. Drain.

4. Mix the dairy-free yogurt, mayonnaise, lemon juice, chives, basil and anchovies in a blender. Season with salt and pepper.
5. Mix the crabmeat, half of the avocado and about 1 tablespoon of the yogurt dressing in a bowl.
6. Mix the romaine, croutons, haricots verts and the remaining avocado with the remaining dressing in another bowl.
7. Prepare the romaine salad among plates and top with the tomatoes.
8. Place some of the crab mixture in the center.

3.3. Snack: Bagel Chips

Yield: 6 to 8 Serving

Ingredients

4 unsliced bagels

2 T. olive oil

Salt and pepper

Instructions

1. Pre-heat the oven to 325 F.
2. Slice the bagels into chips about 1/4" thick.
3. Spread the bagel pieces on an ungreased baking sheet.
4. Lightly brush the pieces with the olive oil and salt and pepper.
5. Bake for 15-20 minutes, flipping half-way through, or until crisp and golden brown.

3.4. Dinner: Jerk Skewers with Black Beans & Rice

Yield: 4 Servings

Ingredients

400g pork fillets, cut into 4cm chunks

2 tbsp. jerk or Creole seasoning

1 tsp ground allspice

1 tbsp. hot chili sauce, plus extra to serve (optional)

3 limes, zest and juice 1, other 2 cut into wedges to serve

½ small pineapple, peeled, cored and cut into 4cm chunks

1 tbsp. vegetable oil

200g basmati rice

400g can black beans, drained and rinsed

Instructions

1. Intermix together the pork, jerk seasoning, allspice, and chili sauce.
2. Thread the pork and pineapple onto the skewers and brush with oil.
3. Cook rice following packaging instructions.
4. Drain, then add back in the saucepan with the beans, stir and keep warm on low.
5. Heat a griddle pan till hot.
6. Cook the skewers for 3 minutes on each side until the pork is cooked through.

7. Serve skewers with the beans and rice, extra chili sauce, if you prefer, and lime wedges.

3.5. Dessert: Non-Dairy Chocolate Ice Cream

Yield: 6 Servings

Ingredients

3 cups unsweetened almond milk

6 large egg yolks

3/4 cup sugar

1/3 cup quality, unsweetened cocoa powder (such as Dutch process)

1/4 tsp xanthan gum, for thickening

1.5 tsp pure vanilla extract

Instructions

1. Add in cocoa powder and half of the almond milk to a saucepan over mid-heat and whisk to combine.
2. Include the remaining almond milk and bring the mixture to a simmer while occasionally.
3. Remove from heat after 2-3 minutes.
4. In a bowl, add the egg yolks and mix until they lighten in color.
5. Gradually add the sugar in small increments while mixing so the two emulsify.
6. You should achieve a ribboning effect - the mixture will form a ribbon when held from the whisk over the bowl.

7. Scoop in roughly 1/3 cup of the warm chocolate-almond milk mixture and mix to combine, in order to temper the eggs.

8. Add the remaining liquid slowly until completely combined.

9. Add in the xanthan gum to the mixture through a sifter and mix once more to help the ice cream thicken.

10. Add the vanilla extract and stir once more.

11. Cover up and refrigerate overnight, or 6-8 hours until cooled.

12. Also chill your ice cream maker canister overnight.

13. Pour the mixture into the pre-chilled ice cream container and prepare according to manufacturer's instructions for approximately 20-30 minutes.

14. Consume as "soft serve" or freeze for 6-8 hours in a freezer-safe container to harden.

Day 2

4.1. Breakfast: Turkey Sausage Patties

Yield: 4-6 Servings

<u>Ingredients</u>

1 lb. ground turkey

1 teaspoon salt

2 teaspoons sage

1 teaspoon fennel seed

1 teaspoon thyme

1 teaspoon black pepper

1/2 teaspoon white pepper

1/2 teaspoon cayenne

1/4 teaspoon garlic powder

1/8 teaspoon ground cloves

1/8 teaspoon nutmeg

1/8 teaspoon allspice

<u>Instructions</u>

1. Add together all ingredients and mix well.
2. Make the patties and cook until browned.
3. Remove from the heat as soon as they're no longer pink inside.
4. Serve up with eggs or a slice of toast.

4.2. Lunch: Mango Chicken Wraps

Yield: 4 Servings

Ingredients

2 (6-ounce) skinless, boneless chicken breast halves

1 tablespoon curry powder

1/4 teaspoon kosher salt

1/2 teaspoon freshly ground black pepper, divided

1 tablespoon olive oil

1/2 cup 2% non-dairy yogurt

1/4 cup mango chutney

3 tablespoons sliced green onions

1 (8.8-ounce) package white naan bread

2 cups mixed spring greens

Instructions

1. Position chicken between 2 sheets of plastic wrap.
2. Pound the chicken to 1/2-inch thickness using a meat mallet or small heavy skillet.
3. Slice each chicken breast half in half crosswise.
4. Add curry powder, salt, and 1/4 teaspoon pepper.
5. Add curry mixture over both sides of the chicken.
6. Heat up a large nonstick skillet over mid-high heat.
7. Add oil; swirl to coat.
8. Add the chicken to the pan.

9. Cook for 3 minutes on each side or until fully done.
10. Remove from pan; let stand 5 minutes.
11. Combine the non-dairy yogurt, chutney, green onions, and remaining 1/4 teaspoon pepper in a bowl.
12. Warm naan according to the packaging directions then cut in half crosswise.
13. Slice the chicken into 1/2-inch-thick slices.
14. Add yogurt mixture over naan halves, spread evenly.
15. Top with greens and cooked chicken then roll up.

4.3. Snack: Baked Corn Dog Bites

Yield: 48 Servings

Ingredients

1 cup fine cornmeal

1 cup all-purpose flour

2 T. dark brown sugar

1 ½ t. baking powder

½ t. baking soda

½ t. salt

1 ¼ cup almond milk

1 large egg, lightly beaten

2 t. olive oil

16 hot dogs or soy dogs, cut into thirds

Instructions

1. Pre-heat oven to 400 F.
2. Line a large baking sheet with parchment paper and place aside.
3. In a mid-sized mixing bowl, sift together the cornmeal, flour, sugar, baking powder, baking soda and salt, and make a funnel in the center.
4. In another bowl, mix together the almond milk, the egg and the oil.

5. Add to the funnel in the dry ingredients and mix until combined.
6. Insert a toothpick or small skewer into each of the hot dog thirds.
7. Dip each hot dog into the batter, turning to coat, and place on the prepared sheet.
8. Bake for 15 to 20 minutes until puffed and golden brown.

4.4. Dinner: Pumpkin Curry with Chickpeas

Yield: 4 Servings

Ingredients

1 tbsp. sunflower oil

3 tbsp. Thai yellow curry paste, or vegetarian alternative

2 onions, finely chopped

3 large stalks lemongrass, bashed with the back of a knife

6 cardamom pods

1 tbsp. mustard seed

1 piece pumpkin or a small squash (about 1kg)

250ml vegetable stock

400ml can reduced-fat coconut milk

400g can chickpeas, drained and rinsed

2 limes

Large handful mint leaves

Naan bread, to serve

Instructions

1. Heat the oil in a small pan.
2. Gently fry the curry paste with the onions, lemongrass, cardamom and mustard seed for 2-3 minutes.
3. Stir the pumpkin or squash into the pan and coat in the paste, then pour in the stock and coconut milk.

4. Bring to a simmer and add the chickpeas, then cook for approximately 10 minutes until the pumpkin is tender.
5. Squeeze the juice of one lime into the curry.
6. Slice the additional lime into wedges to serve alongside.
7. Tear over mint leaves just before serving with warm naan bread and slices lime wedges.

4.5. Dessert: Dairy-Free Chocolate Chip Cookie Dough Ice Cream

Yield: 6 Servings

Ingredients

1 batch chocolate chip cookie dough frozen into balls, and then chopped into small pieces

3 cups full-fat canned coconut milk

1/2 cup maple syrup or raw honey

Pinch of Celtic sea salt

1 tablespoon vanilla extract

Instructions

1. Mix jointly coconut milk, maple syrup, salt and vanilla.
2. Freeze in an ice cream maker according to the manufacturer's instructions.
3. After freezing, take away the blade and add in the cookie dough and stir.
4. Serve up.

Day 3

5.1. Breakfast: French Toast

Yield: 2 Servings

<u>Ingredients</u>

4 slices gluten free bread

2 medium eggs

2 tablespoons orange juice

1/4 cup almond milk (plain or vanilla) or 1/4 cup rice milk (plain or vanilla) or 1/4 cup soymilk (plain or vanilla)

1/4 teaspoon cinnamon

1/8 teaspoon nutmeg

1/4 teaspoon salt

1/4 teaspoon vanilla extract

2 tablespoons ghee or 2 tablespoons dairy-free margarine

<u>Optional</u>

2 teaspoons honey

<u>Ingredients</u>

1. Mix together all the ingredients except the ghee or dairy-free margarine.
2. Add the bread in a pie pan or small baking dish until blended.
3. Heat ghee, or dairy-free margarine in non-stick pan or griddle over mid-high heat.
4. If you're using a dense bread, allow it to soak for 3-5 minutes on each side.

5. If you're utilizing a homemade bread or a softer bread, soak for only 1-2 minutes on each side.
6. Utilizing a fork or tongs, take away each slice of bread from the liquid and allow excess liquid to drip off.
7. Place in hot ghee or dairy- free margarine and cook on each side until browned.
8. Serve up immediately with your choice of maple syrup, jam, or fresh fruit.

5.2. Lunch: Grilled Hummus and Vegetable Wrap

Yield: 4 Servings

<u>Ingredients</u>

2 medium zucchini, cut lengthwise into 1/4-inch slices
2 teaspoons olive oil
1/8 teaspoon salt
Pinch freshly ground black pepper
1 cup store-bought hummus
4 pieces whole-wheat wrap bread (about 9 inches in diameter)
1/4 cup pine nuts, toasted
1 medium red bell pepper, thinly sliced
2 ounces baby spinach leaves (2 cups lightly packed)
1/2 cup red onion thinly sliced into half moons
1/4 cup fresh mint leaves

<u>Instructions</u>

1. Pre-heat the grill or grill pan over mid-heat.
2. Apply oil to both sides of the zucchini slices and sprinkle with the salt and pepper.
3. Grill until tender and slightly browned for approximately 4 minutes each side.
4. Spread 1/4 cup of the hummus over each piece of wrap bread.
5. Apply 1 tablespoon of pine nuts on top.

6. Add on top the 3 slices of zucchini, 2 pieces of red pepper, 1/2 cup of the spinach, a few sliced onions, and 1 tablespoon of the mint.
7. Roll up and cut in half diagonally.

5.3. Snack: Crispy Apple Bites

Yield: 16 Servings

<u>Ingredients</u>

1 apple

<u>Instructions</u>

1. Prepare oven to 284 F.
2. Thinly slice the apple through the core.
3. Arrange the slices on a baking tray lined with parchment and bake for 40 minutes.
4. Cool until crisp.

5.4. Dinner: Lemon Zest Spaghetti with Tuna & Broccoli

Yield: 4 Servings

Ingredients

350g spaghetti

250g broccoli, cut into small florets

2 shallots, finely chopped

85g pitted green olives, halved

2 tbsp. capers, drained

198g can tuna in oil

Zest and juice 1 lemon

1 tbsp. olive oil, plus extra for drizzling

Instructions

1. Boil spaghetti for 6 minutes in lightly salted water.
2. Place in the broccoli and boil for 4 minutes more or until both tender.
3. Mix the shallots, olives, capers, tuna and lemon zest and juice in a bowl.
4. Drain the pasta and broccoli.
5. Add to the bowl and toss really well with olive oil and black pepper.
6. Serve with extra olive oil drizzled over.

5.5. Dessert: Scrumptious Banana Cookies

Yield: 36 Servings

<u>Ingredients</u>

3 ripe bananas

2 cups rolled oats

1 cup dates, pitted and chopped

1/3 cup vegetable oil

1 teaspoon vanilla extract

<u>Instructions</u>

1. Pre-heat the oven to 350 F.
2. In a bowl, mash the bananas.
3. Add in oats, dates, oil, vanilla and stir.
4. Mix well, and let sit for 15 minutes.
5. Drop teaspoonfuls onto an un-greased cookie sheet.
6. Bake for 20 minutes or until lightly brown.

Day 4

6.1. Breakfast: Baked Blueberry-Apple Oatmeal

Yield: 2 Servings

Ingredients

2 cups quick-cooking oats

1 cup rolled oats

1/2 cup packed brown sugar

2 t. baking powder

1/2 t. cinnamon

3/4 t. salt

1/4 t. ground ginger

3 T. flax meal (finely ground flax seeds)

1/4 cup warm water

1 cup almond milk or soy milk

1/3 cup maple syrup

1/4 cup melted soy dairy- free margarine

1/2 cup fresh blueberries

1/3 cup chopped peeled apples

Instructions

1. Prepare the oven to 350 F.
2. Lightly oil or grease an 8" square baking pan.
3. In a bowl, mix together the quick-cooking oats, rolled oats, brown sugar, baking powder, cinnamon, salt and ginger and place aside.

4. In another bowl, combine the flax meal with the warm water until the mixture is a bit goopy looking and place aside.

5. In an additional mixing bowl add together the almond milk, maple syrup and melted soy dairy- free margarine.

6. Add in to the dry ingredients along with the flax mixture. Stir until combined.

7. Fold in the blueberries and apples.

8. Spread the mixture in the prepared pan and bake for 35-40 minutes.

9. Cut into 8 squares and serve up warm with almond milk or soy milk.

6.2. Lunch: Chicken Fried Rice

<u>Ingredients</u>

2 tablespoons dark sesame oil

1 tablespoon canola oil

1 cup chopped carrot

1 cup coarsely chopped broccoli florets

1 cup diced skinless, boneless rotisserie chicken breast

1 cup frozen petite green peas

2/3 cup sliced green onions (4 green onions), divided

2 garlic cloves, minced

1 teaspoon grated peeled fresh ginger

3 cups cooked long-grain brown rice, chilled

2 large eggs, lightly beaten

2 tablespoons lower-sodium soy sauce

1/2 teaspoon kosher salt

1/4 teaspoon freshly ground black pepper

<u>Instructions</u>

1. Heat a nonstick skillet over mid-high heat.
2. Add in oils then swirl to coat.
3. Include carrot and broccoli then stir-fry 3 minutes or until crisp-tender.
4. Place in chicken, peas, 1/2 cup onions, garlic, and ginger.
5. Stir-fry for 2 minutes or until onions are tender.

6. Add in the rice and cook 3 minutes or until thoroughly heated. Stir occasionally.
7. Reduce heat to medium temperature.
8. Push rice mixture to one side of the pan.
9. Add the eggs to the opposite side of pan.
10. Allow to cook for 10 seconds without stirring.
11. Allow to cook for an additional 2 minutes or until eggs are scrambled.
12. Add in the soy sauce, salt, and pepper.
13. Sprinkle with remaining onions.
14. Serve.

6.3. Snack: Bean and Chili Dip

Yield: 4 Servings

<u>Ingredients</u>

395g can kidney beans in chili sauce

400g can mixed beans, drained

326g can sweetcorn, drained

Small red onion, chopped

1 red chili, deseeded and chopped

Small bunch coriander, chopped

350g vegetable sticks and tortilla chips, to serve

<u>Instructions</u>

1. Blend three-quarters of the kidney beans and half the mixed beans until smooth.
2. Add into a bowl and add the remaining ingredients with some seasoning.
3. Serve with vegetable sticks or tortilla chips for dipping.

6.4. Dinner: Blackened Tuna Steaks with Mango Salsa

Yield: 4 Servings

Ingredients

2 tablespoons olive oil

2 tablespoons lime juice

2 cloves garlic, minced

4 tuna steaks

1 fresh mango - peeled, pitted, and chopped

1/4 cup finely chopped red bell pepper

1/2 Spanish onion, finely chopped

1 green onion, chopped

2 tablespoons chopped fresh cilantro

1 jalapeno pepper, seeded and minced

2 tablespoons lime juice

1 1/2 teaspoons olive oil

2 tablespoons paprika

1 tablespoon cayenne pepper

1 tablespoon onion powder

2 teaspoons salt

1 teaspoon ground black pepper

1 teaspoon dried thyme

1 teaspoon dried basil

1 teaspoon dried oregano

1 tablespoon garlic powder

4 tablespoons olive oil

Instructions

1. Mix the olive oil, lime juice, and garlic.
2. Rub the tuna steaks with the mixture.
3. Place the steaks in a sealable container and chill in refrigerator for 3 hours.
4. Mix the mango, bell pepper, Spanish onion, green onion, cilantro, and jalapeno pepper in a bowl and stir.
5. Add the lime juice and 1 1/2 teaspoons olive oil and combine.
6. Chill in the refrigerator for 1 hour.
7. Blend together the paprika, cayenne pepper, onion powder, salt, pepper, thyme, basil, oregano, and garlic powder in a bowl.
8. Take out the tuna steaks from the refrigerator and gently rinse with water and then coat each side of each steak in the spice mixture.
9. Heat up 2 tablespoons of olive oil in a large skillet over mid-heat.
10. Lay the tuna steaks into the hot oil.
11. Cook the tuna on one side for 3 minutes then remove.
12. Pour the remaining 2 tablespoons of olive-oil into the skillet and allow it to get hot.
13. Lay the tuna on the uncooked side down into the skillet and cook additional 3 minutes then remove from heat.

14. Spoon about 1/2 cup of the mango salsa onto each of the tuna steaks.
15. Serve.

6.5. Dessert: Ginger Cookies

Yield: 24 Servings

<u>Ingredients</u>

2 1/4 cups all-purpose flour

2 teaspoons ground ginger

1 teaspoon baking soda

3/4 teaspoon ground cinnamon

1/2 teaspoon ground cloves

1/4 teaspoon salt

3/4 cup dairy- free margarine, softened(or oil)

1 cup white sugar

1 egg

1 tablespoon water

1/4 cup molasses

2 tablespoons white sugar

<u>Instructions</u>

1. Pre-heat oven to 350 degrees F.
2. Mix together the flour, ginger, baking soda, cinnamon, cloves, salt and place aside.
3. In a bowl, cream together the dairy- free margarine and 1 cup sugar until light and fluffy.
4. Add in the egg.
5. Mix in the water and molasses.

6. Stir the sifted ingredients into the molasses mixture.
7. Shape the dough into walnut sized balls.
8. Roll them in the remaining 2 tablespoons of sugar.
9. Position the cookies 2 inches apart onto an ungreased cookie sheet, and flatten.
10. Bake for 8 to 10 minutes in the pre-heated oven.
11. Allow the cookies to cool on baking sheet for 5 minutes.

Day 5

7.1. Breakfast: Almond & Cranberry Granola

Yield: 2 Servings

<u>Ingredients</u>

8 cups old-fashioned rolled oats

½ cup ground almonds

½ cup whole or slivered almonds

¾ cup unsalted, raw sunflower seeds

¾ cup raw, shelled pumpkin seeds

½ cup millet

1 t. ground cinnamon

¼ t. ground ginger

¼ t. salt

½ cup maple syrup

½ cup honey

¾ cup canola oil

1 cup dried cranberries

½ cup dried apricots

<u>Instructions</u>

1. Prepare the oven at 300 F.

2. Line a large baking sheet with parchment paper.

3. In a bowl mix oats, almond meal, seeds, almonds, millet, cinnamon, ginger and salt until combined.

4. In another bowl blend together the maple syrup, honey and oil.

5. Mix well together the wet ingredients with the dry in two additions.

6. Spread out the granola evenly onto the prepared sheets and bake for 45-55 minutes.

7. Take away the pans from the oven half-way through and flip the granola gently with a metal spatula.

8. Be sure to rotate the pans to ensure even baking.

9. Remove the pan from the oven when the granola is golden brown.

10. Cool for 20 minutes before folding in the dried fruits.

11. The granola will remain fresh for up to two weeks in an airtight container.

7.2. Lunch: Sweet and Sour Chicken

Yield: 4 Servings

Ingredients

3 tablespoons all-purpose flour

1/2 teaspoon garlic powder

1/2 teaspoon salt

1/2 teaspoon ground black pepper

1 pound skinless, boneless chicken

Breast halves, cut into 1-inch cubes

3 tablespoons vegetable oil, divided

3 celery ribs, sliced

2 green bell peppers, diced

1 onion, chopped

1/2 cup ketchup

1/2 cup lemon juice

1/2 cup crushed pineapple with syrup

1/3 cup packed brown sugar

Instructions

1. Mix together the flour, garlic powder, salt, and black pepper in a bowl
2. Roll up and coat chicken cubes in flour mix.
3. Warm up 2 tablespoons vegetable oil in a skillet over mid-high temperature.
4. Prepare and stir chicken in hot oil until no longer pink in the center and juices run clear, 8 to 10 minutes then place aside.

5. Warm up 1 tablespoon of vegetable oil in the same skillet over mid-heat.
6. Cook and stir collectively the celery, green peppers, and onion in a heated oil until tender for approximately 5 minutes.
7. Return the chicken to the skillet.
8. Whisk together ketchup, lemon juice, pineapple, and brown sugar in a bowl.
9. Add to the skillet and bring to boil.
10. Stir chicken and vegetables in sauce till heated through for approximately 2 to 3 minutes.

7.3. Snack: Curry Potato Wedges

Yield: 6 Servings

Ingredients

6 large baking potatoes
1 tbsp. olive oil
2 tbsp. tikka masala curry paste
1 tbsp. tomato purée
400g can reduced-fat coconut milk
Handful coriander leaves, chopped (optional)
Juice ½ lemon

Instructions

1. Heat the oven to 350 F.
2. Cut the potatoes into wedges.
3. Apply the oil into a sizeable pan.
4. Add in the wedges until coated and season with pepper.
5. Bake for approximately 35-40 minutes until golden.
6. Place the curry paste and tomato purée in a saucepan.
7. Mix and fry for 1 min.
8. Include the coconut milk then boil.
9. Turn down and simmer for 10 minutes.
10. Season and finish with a drizzle of lemon juice and a scattering of coriander.

7.4. Dinner: Sweet and Spicy Chicken

Yield: 4 Servings

<u>Ingredients</u>

1 tablespoon brown sugar

2 tablespoons honey

1/4 cup soy sauce

2 teaspoons chopped fresh ginger root

2 teaspoons chopped garlic

2 tablespoons hot sauce

Salt and pepper to taste

4 skinless, boneless chicken breast

Halves - cut into 1/2 inch strips

1 tablespoon vegetable oil

<u>Instructions</u>

1. Mix well the brown sugar, honey, soy sauce, ginger, garlic and hot sauce in a bowl.
2. Lightly salt and pepper the chicken strips.
3. Heat up the oil in a large skillet over mid-heat.
4. Add in the chicken strips and brown on both sides, approximately 1 minute per side.
5. Distribute the sauce over the chicken.
6. Simmer, then uncover until the sauce thickens for about 8 to 10 minutes.

7.5. Dessert: Apple Enchilada

Yield: 6 Servings

Ingredients

1 (21 ounce) can apple pie filling

6 (8 inch) flour tortillas

1 teaspoon ground cinnamon

1/3 cup dairy- free margarine

1/2 cup white sugar

1/2 cup packed brown sugar

1/2 cup water

Instructions

1. Pre-heat the oven to 350 F.
2. Spoon the fruit evenly onto all tortillas sprinkle and with cinnamon.
3. Roll up tortillas and place seam side down on a lightly greased 8x8 baking pan.
4. Bring the dairy- free margarine, sugars and water to boil in a mid-sized sauce pan.
5. Turn down the heat and simmer, stirring constantly for 3 minutes.
6. Distribute the sauce over tortillas then sprinkle with extra cinnamon on top if preferred.
7. Bake in a pre-heated oven for 20 minutes.

Day 6

8.1. Breakfast: Toasted Peanut Butter and Banana Sandwich

Yield: 1 Serving

Ingredients

2 slices granary bread

1 small banana

½ tsp cinnamon

1 tbsp. crunchy peanut butter

Instructions

1. Toast the bread.
2. Slice the banana.
3. Layer the banana on one slice of toast and slightly sprinkle with cinnamon.
4. Apply the second slice of bread with the peanut butter.
5. Place the bottom and the top pf the sandwich the together and serve.

8.2. Lunch: Chicken Fajitas

Yield: 2 Servings

<u>Ingredients</u>

1 tablespoon chili powder

1 teaspoon cumin

1 teaspoon paprika

1/4 teaspoon cayenne pepper

1/4 teaspoon garlic powder

1 teaspoon salt

1 teaspoon ground black pepper

3 tablespoons olive oil, divided

1 1/2 pounds boneless, skinless chicken breast, sliced into strips

2 bell peppers, stem and core removed, sliced

1 onion, thinly sliced

8 small tortillas

Optional Toppings:
Fresh cilantro, chopped

Tomatoes, diced

Dairy-Free cheddar cheese, shredded

Avocado, sliced

Vegan sour cream or non-dairy yogurt

<u>Instructions</u>

Fajita Seasoning:

1. Combine together the chili powder, cumin, paprika, cayenne pepper, garlic powder, salt, and pepper in a bowl and place aside.
2. Heat up 1 tablespoon of olive-oil in a pan over mid-high heat.
3. Add in the strips of chicken to the pan then sprinkle with 3/4 of the fajita seasoning.
4. Mix well and cook for 6 to 10 minutes or until browned.
5. In another pan, heat the remaining oil over mid heat.
6. Add in the peppers and onions.
7. Stir in the remaining fajita seasoning.
8. Cook until the vegetables are soft for approximately 8 to 10 minutes. Stir occasionally.
9. Meanwhile, wrap the stack of tortillas in tin foil and warm in a 250 degree oven.
10. Assemble the fajitas by filling the warmed tortillas with a mix of chicken, peppers and onions.
11. Top with your favorite garnishes.

8.3. Snack: Garlic & Rosemary Bites

Yield: 4 Servings

Ingredients

4 large potatoes, thinly sliced

3 tbsp. olive oil

2 garlic cloves, sliced

1 tbsp. rosemary needles

Instructions

1. Heat up the oven to medium heat and simmer the potatoes in salted water for 3 minutes.
2. Drain well, tip into a shallow baking tray.
3. Toss with the oil, garlic, rosemary and seasoning.
4. Position pieces in one layer and bake for 10-15 minutes or until crisp and golden.

8.4. Dinner: Pineapple Chicken Strips

Yield: 10 Servings

Ingredients

1 cup pineapple juice

1/2 cup packed brown sugar

1/3 cup light soy sauce

2 pounds chicken breast tenderloins or strips

Skewers

Instructions

1. Over medium heat, mix pineapple juice, brown sugar, and soy sauce.
2. Remove from heat before boil.
3. Place chicken tenders in a bowl and cover with the pineapple marinade.
4. Refrigerate for 30 minutes.
5. Pre-heat grill at mid-heat.
6. Thread chicken onto wooden skewers.
7. Lightly oil the grill.
8. Grill chicken tenders 5 minutes on each side.
9. Serve.

8.5. Dessert: Vanilla Vegan Cake

Yield: 6-9 Servings

<u>Ingredients</u>

1 1/2 cups unbleached all-purpose flour

1 cup sugar

1 teaspoon baking soda

1/2 teaspoon salt

1/2 cup vegetable oil

1 cup soymilk

1 tablespoon vanilla extract

1 tablespoon vinegar

<u>Instructions</u>

1. Heat oven to 350 F.
2. Line an 8-inch round or square cake pan with parchment paper.
3. Grease bottom and sides of the pan.
4. Flour the pan.
5. Mix then flour, sugar, baking soda, and salt.
6. Add in vegetable oil, soy milk, and vanilla extract; whisk until no lumps appear and batter is smooth.
7. Include in vinegar, stir about seven times, and quickly pour into pan.
8. Bake for approximately 30 minutes.
9. Check until cake begins to pull away from sides.

10. Let sit for ten to 15 minutes, and allow to cool.

Day7

9.1. Breakfast: Tropical Breakfast Smoothie

Yield: 2-3 Servings

Ingredients

3 passion fruits

1 banana, chopped

1 small mango, peeled, stoned and chopped

300ml orange juice

Ice cubes

Instructions

1. Scoop out the pulp of the passion fruits and add into a blender.
2. Place in the banana, mango and orange juice.
3. Blend well until smooth and serve.
4. Top the drink with ice cubes if preferred.

9.2. Lunch: Turkey Chipotle Chili

Yield: 4 Servings

Ingredients

2 tablespoons olive oil

1 1/2 pounds ground turkey

3 large carrots, chopped

5-6 stalks celery, chopped

1 onion, chopped

4 cloves garlic, minced

Salt

Pepper

2 heaping tablespoons finely chopped canned chipotle chilies in adobo

1 can (15 ounces) tomato sauce

1 1/2 cups chicken stock

2 cups blue corn tortilla chips (optional)

1 cup shredded vegan cheese (optional)

Instructions

1. Heat olive oil over medium-high heat.
2. Add in the turkey and cook until browned.
3. Add in the carrots, celery, onion, and garlic.
4. Cook for approximately 10 minutes until soft.
5. Combine chipotle sauce and chilies with tomato sauce.

6. Add to vegetables with broth and boil.
7. Reduce temperature and simmer until thickened.
8. Turn on broiler.
9. Move the chili to a casserole dish and top with chips and cheese, if preferred.
10. Broil for a few minutes until cheese melts.

9.3. Snack: Spring Rolls with Ginger Sauce

Yield: 6 Servings

Ingredients

6 rice-paper wrappers

2 cups radish sprouts (1/2 ounce)

1 red beet, trimmed and thinly sliced crosswise

1 medium carrot, peeled and julienned

1 cucumber, julienned

1 red bell pepper, stem and seeds removed, julienned

3/4 cup coarsely grated daikon

3 medium carrots, peeled and coarsely chopped

1 small shallot, quartered

2 tablespoons coarsely grated peeled fresh ginger

1/4 cup rice-wine vinegar (not seasoned)

2 tablespoons low-sodium soy sauce

1/4 teaspoon toasted sesame oil

Pinch each of coarse salt and freshly ground pepper

1/4 cup vegetable oil

1/4 cup water

Instructions

Prepare the spring rolls:
1. Soak one rice-paper wrapper in a bowl of hot water until flexible.
2. Transfer over to a flat working surface.

3. Position 1/6 of the sprouts, beet slices, carrot, cucumber, bell pepper, and daikon on the wrapper, towards the bottom of the rice paper.
4. Fold in the ends and roll tightly.
5. Repeat with the remaining ingredients.

Prepare the dipping sauce:

1. Blend well the carrots, shallot, ginger, vinegar, soy sauce, sesame oil, salt, and pepper in a food processor until smooth.
2. Continue to add vegetable oil and then water through the feed tube in a slow and steady.
3. Serve up with spring rolls.

9.4. Dinner: Beef & Veggie Beer Chili

Yield: 4 Servings

<u>Ingredients</u>

1 medium onion, chopped

1 green bell pepper, chopped

Vegetable cooking spray

1/2 pound extra lean minced beef

1 teaspoon finely chopped garlic

2 tablespoons chili powder

2 teaspoons cumin powder

1 teaspoon dried oregano

1 (10 ounce) can chopped tomatoes, undrained

1-3 finely chopped fresh (or preserved) green chilies

1 (14 ounce) can no-salt added kidney beans, drained

1 (14 ounce) can low-salt: beef stock

1 (12 ounce bottle) lager beer

Garnish: Lime wedges, coriander leaf, fat-free sour cream, baked tortilla chips

<u>Instructions</u>

1. Coat a sizable soup pot with cooking spray.
2. Sauté onions and bell pepper over mid-high heat for 3 to 4 minutes or until onions are translucent.

3. Add in minced beef and garlic and cook for approximately 5 minutes.
4. Stir to break up chunks and cook until beef is no longer pink.
5. Drain off any fat.
6. Add in the chili powder, cumin and oregano and cook.
7. Stir constantly for approximately 2 minutes.
8. Include the tomatoes and green chilies and remaining ingredients except the garnishes.
9. Bring to a boil.
10. Reduce the heat and simmer for 20 minutes.
11. Serve up with garnishes.

9.5. Dessert: Pineapple Orange Sorbet

Yield: 10 Servings

<u>Ingredients</u>

1/2 cup water

1/2 cup granulated sugar

2 cups orange juice

1 tablespoon lemon juice

1 (20 ounce) can crushed pineapple

2 teaspoons freshly grated orange zest

<u>Instructions</u>

1. In a mid-sized pan, bring water and sugar to a simmer over mid-high heat until sugar is well dissolved.
2. Puree the pineapple with its juice until smooth in a food processor.
3. Transfer over to a metal bowl, and stir in syrup, lemon juice, orange juice, and orange zest.
4. Freeze the mixture until slightly firm, but not frozen.
5. Blend the mixture again in the food processor or with an electric mixer until smooth.
6. Transfer over to a freezer container and freeze until firm for approximately 2 hours.

Day 8

10.1. Breakfast: Early Sunrise Smoothie

Yield: 2-4 Servings

Ingredients

1 cup (250 mL) silken tofu (such as 1/2 package Vitasoy Silken Tofu)

1/2 medium ripe banana

1/2 cup orange juice

1/4 cup honey (or to taste)

1 scoop protein powder

3/4 cup fresh or frozen strawberries, or fruit of choice

1 cup ice

Ingredients

1. Combine and blend together tofu, banana, orange juice, honey and fruit until smooth.
2. Add in ice then continue to blend until creamy.
3. Serve up immediately.

10.2. Lunch: Smoked Turkey Reuben

Yield: 1 Sandwich

<u>Ingredients</u>

2 tablespoons Dijon mustard

8 slices rye bread

4 (1-ounce) Vegan Swiss cheese slices

8 ounces smoked turkey, thinly sliced

2/3 cup sauerkraut, drained and rinsed

1/4 cup fat-free Thousand Island dressing

1 tablespoon canola oil, divided

<u>Instructions</u>

1. Apply 3/4 teaspoon mustard over each bread.
2. Add 1 cheese slice on each of the 4 bread slices.
3. Separate the turkey evenly over the cheese.
4. Add to each serving 2 1/2 tablespoons sauerkraut and 1 tablespoon dressing.
5. Add each serving with 1 bread slice, mustard sides down.
6. Warm 1 1/2 teaspoons canola oil in a non-stick skillet over medium-high temperature.
7. Add in 2 sandwiches to pan and top with another heavy skillet.
8. Cook for 3 minutes on each side or until golden.
9. Take away sandwiches from pan, and keep warm.

10. Replicate the procedure with the remaining oil and sandwiches.

10.3. Snack: Baked Plantain Chips

Yield: 4 Servings

Ingredients

2 pounds plantains or green bananas, scored, peeled, and thinly sliced on the diagonal

1/4 cup vegetable oil

Coarse salt and ground pepper

Instructions

1. Pre-heat the oven to 350 F, with the racks on the upper and lower thirds.
2. Divide the plantains between two rimmed baking sheets.
3. Toss with oil.
4. Position in a single layer on the sheets.
5. Season lightly with salt and pepper.
6. Bake until golden and crispy for approximately, 30 to 35 minutes, rotating sheets and flipping plantains halfway through.
7. Pat dry the plantains on paper towels.

10.4. Dinner: Red Whine Beef and Mushroom Sauté

Yield: 4 Servings

Ingredients

1 pound boneless beef sirloin steak (3/4 inch thick)

1 teaspoon black pepper, freshly cracked

1/4 teaspoon sea salt

2 teaspoons vegetable oil, divided

1/2 cup button mushrooms, sliced

1/2 cup Portobello mushrooms, sliced

1/2 cup shiitake mushrooms, sliced

1/2 cup dry red wine

1 cup low-sodium beef broth

Instructions

1. Massage the steak with pepper and salt.
2. Heat up 1 teaspoon oil an oven-proof skillet over mid-high heat.
3. Add the steak and cook for 4 minutes.
4. Place the skillet in a 450°F oven and bake for approximately 4 minutes for medium-rare, or until meat reaches desired likeness.
5. Remove from skillet and allow it to stand for 10 minutes.
6. In the same skillet, heat the remaining oil over mid-high heat.
7. Add in the mushrooms and cook until golden brown.

8. Add in the wine and bring to a boil.
9. Simmer until the liquid reduces by half.
10. Place in the broth and simmer until reduced by half again.
11. When serving, thinly slice steak and top with the mushroom sauce.

10.5. Dessert: Homemade Dairy-Free Peach Ice Cream

Yield: 6 Servings

Ingredients

4 cups fresh peaches or 1 lb. frozen peaches, sliced
1 cup light vanilla soymilk
3/4 cup light brown sugar, packed
2 tablespoons lemon juice
1/2 teaspoon vanilla extract
1/2 teaspoon salt

Instructions

1. Spread peach slices in baking dish and freeze for approximately 4 hours or until solid.
2. Add the peaches and the remaining ingredients in a food processor.
3. Blend well until smooth.
4. Serve up immediately or freeze for up to 30 minutes for a firm texture.

Day 9

11.1. Breakfast: Banana, Granola, Chocolate Chip Muffins

Yield: 16 Muffins

<u>Ingredients</u>

Banana Muffins:

2-1/2 cups gluten-free flour mix (ingredients below)

1 cup brown sugar, loosely packed

1-1/2 teaspoons baking soda

1-1/2 teaspoons baking powder

1 teaspoon xanthan gum, guar gum, or agar powder

½ teaspoon ground cinnamon

½ teaspoon salt

2 cups mashed, extremely ripe bananas (about 5-6 bananas)

½ cup grapeseed, canola, or sunflower oil

Water, room temperature

1 tablespoon vanilla extract

2 cups dairy-free chocolate chips

2 cups dairy-free, gluten-free granola

Homemade Gluten-Free Flour Blend:

1 cup buckwheat flour

1 cup brown rice flour

¾ cup tapioca starch/flour

¼ cup amaranth flour

½ cup sorghum, teff, or quinoa flour

Instructions

1. Pre-heat your oven to 350°F.
2. Line the 16 muffin cups with paper liners then oil lightly.
3. In a bowl, intermix the flour mix, brown sugar, baking soda, baking powder, gum, cinnamon, and salt.
4. In another bowl, combine together the bananas, oil, water, and vanilla.
5. Include the wet ingredients to the dry ingredients and gently stir until the batter is uniform and smooth.
6. Add in the chocolate chips.
7. Utilizing a half-cup measuring, scoop the batter into the prepared muffin tins.
8. Sprinkle the granola over the tops of the muffins.
9. Bake for approximately 25 to 30 minutes, or until a toothpick comes out dry.
10. Serve up or keep in airtight container.

11.2. Lunch: Spicy Chicken Pitas

Yield: 4 Servings

<u>Ingredients</u>

1 pound boneless, skinless chicken breasts, trimmed

1 1/2 teaspoons garam masala, (see Tip), divided

3/4 teaspoon kosher salt, divided

1 cup thinly sliced seeded cucumber

3/4 cup non-dairy yogurt

1 tablespoon chopped fresh cilantro, or mint

2 teaspoons lemon juice

Freshly ground pepper, to taste

4 6-inch whole-wheat pitas, warmed

1 cup shredded romaine lettuce

2 small or 1 large tomato, sliced

1/4 cup thinly sliced red onion

<u>Instructions</u>

1. Pre-heat grill to mid-high or position rack in upper third of oven and pre-heat broiler.
2. Oil the grill rack if broiling, coat a broiler pan with cooking spray.
3. Apply 1 teaspoon garam masala and 1/2 teaspoon salt to the chicken.

4. Position the chicken on the grill rack or the prepared pan and cook until no longer pink in the middle.
5. Move the chicken to a clean cutting board and allow to rest for 5 minutes.
6. Combine the cucumber, non-dairy yogurt, cilantro (or mint), lemon juice, the remaining 1/2 teaspoon garam masala and 1/4 teaspoon salt and pepper in a bowl.
7. Slice the chicken in thin pieces.
8. Split open the warm pitas and fill with the chicken, yogurt sauce, lettuce, tomato and onion.
9. Serve.

11.3. Snack: Tossed Edamame with Chile Salt

Yield: 4 Servings

Ingredients

1/2 teaspoon crushed red-pepper flakes

1 tablespoon coarse salt

1/2 teaspoon sugar

1 pound frozen edamame in shells

Instructions

1. Grind the red-pepper flakes in a spice grinder.
2. Apply with salt and sugar in a bowl.
3. Set a large pot of water to boil.
4. Add in the frozen edamame, and cook until bright green and heated through, for approximately 4 minutes.
5. Drain and transfer to a bowl.
6. Apply with chili-salt mixture.
7. Serve.

11.4. Dinner: Chicken and Squash Casserole

Yield: 4 Servings

Ingredients

1 clove garlic, minced

1/2 teaspoon minced fresh rosemary + 2 whole sprigs

1 1/2 teaspoons minced fresh thyme + 2 whole sprigs

1 teaspoon salt, divided

2 1/2 tablespoons olive oil, divided

1 1/4 pounds boneless, skinless chicken thighs

1/2 pound carrots, cut into small, 1/2 inch pieces

1/2 pound zucchini, sliced into 1/4 inch coins

1/2 pound summer squash, sliced into 1/4 inch coins

1 small red onion, cut into wedges

Instructions

1. Pre-heat oven to 350 F.
2. In a bowl, combine together garlic, minced rosemary, minced thyme, 1/2 teaspoon salt and 1 1/2 tablespoons olive oil.
3. Massage mixture all over the chicken thighs and place aside.
4. Toss carrots, zucchini, summer squash and red onions with leftover 1/2 teaspoon salt and 1 tablespoon olive oil then scatter on the bottom of a sizable baking dish.

5. Tuck the sprigs of rosemary and thyme underneath the vegetables, then position the chicken thighs over the vegetables.
6. Bake in the oven for 30 minutes, or until chicken reaches 165 F.
7. Serve.

11.5. Dessert: Fruit Ice Cream

Yield: 6 Servings

<u>Ingredients</u>

2 large bananas, ripe, peeled

1 medium avocado, ripe, peeled, pitted

2 cups frozen strawberries or 2 cups frozen cherries

<u>Instructions</u>

1. Apply all ingredients into a blender or food processor and puree.
2. Add sweetener such as agave nectar, to taste.
3. Place in freezer-safe bowl with lid and freeze.
4. Serve.

Day 10

12.1. Breakfast: Delightful Danish Puffs

Yield: 2 puffs

<u>Ingredients</u>

For the crust:

1 cup all-purpose flour
½ teaspoon salt
Coconut oil
2-4 tablespoons cold water

For the puff:

½ cup coconut oil
1 cup water
1 cup all-purpose flour
1 teaspoon almond extract
3 eggs

For the frosting:

1 tablespoon coconut oil, melted
1 ½ cups powdered sugar
2 tablespoons of Coconut Milk Beverage or Almond Milk
1 teaspoon almond extract

Additional:

½ cup chopped almonds

Instructions

Preparing the Crust:

1. Mix the flour and salt in a bowl.
2. Add in coconut oil using a pastry blender.
3. Include 2 tablespoons of cold water.
4. Stir utilizing a fork until dough shapes into a ball. Add more water if necessary.
5. Chill in the fridge for one hour.
6. Separate the dough in half.
7. Press each half into a 12" X 3" rectangle shape on an ungreased cookie sheet.

Preparing the Puff:

1. In a 2 quart pan, combine ½ cup coconut oil and 1 cup water. Let boil.
2. Take away from heat.
3. Stir in 1 cup flour and 1 teaspoon almond extract.
4. Add in eggs and beat with a wooden spoon till smooth and glossy.
5. Spread half of the topping over every rectangle shape of dough.
6. Bake in the oven for 45-50 minutes in a pre-heated 350 F oven, till golden brown.
7. Cool for 10 minutes.

Preparing the Frosting:

1. Mix melted coconut oil, powdered sugar, coconut (or almond) milk, and almond extract in a bowl and stir well to combine.
2. Apply more coconut (or almond) milk if needed to make a spreadable frosting.
3. Apply the frosting over slightly warm puffs.
4. Drizzle with chopped almonds.

12.2. Lunch: Ham and Cheese Turnovers

Yield: 4 Servings

Ingredients

1 1-pound package refrigerated pizza dough
8 ounces deli ham, thinly sliced
4 ounces Vegan Swiss cheese, thinly sliced
1/2 yellow onion, cut into thin rings
2 teaspoons whole-grain mustard
2 tablespoons extra-virgin olive oil
1 small head romaine, torn into pieces

Instructions

1. Heat up the oven to 400 F.
2. Roll up the pizza dough into a 14-inch circle then cut into 8 triangles shapes.
3. Apply a slice of ham and cheese and some onion on the end of each triangle and roll the dough up around the filling.
4. Move the rolls to a parchment-lined baking sheet.
5. Bake in the oven till golden and crisp, approximately 20 minutes.
6. Intermix the mustard and oil in a bowl and toss with the romaine.
7. Serve up along with the turnovers.

12.3. Snack: Popcorn Balls

Yield: 10 Servings

Ingredients

1 tablespoon canola oil

3 tablespoons un-popped popcorn kernels

2 tablespoons unsalted butter

2 1/4 cups mini marshmallows

1 cup honey-nut toasted oat cereal

1 ounce pretzel sticks, broken into pieces

1/4 cup chopped dry-roasted peanuts, salted

Instructions

1. Heat up the oil in pan over medium-high temperature.
2. Add kernels then cover and cook 4 minutes, shaking the pan frequently.
3. Whenever the popping slows, remove pan from heat then allow to stand.
4. Melt the butter in a pan over mid-heat.
5. Add in marshmallows then cook for 2 minutes.
6. Take away from heat.
7. Apply 3 cups popcorn and the remaining ingredients and stir.
8. Cool down for 2 minutes.
9. Shape into 10 (3-inch) balls.

10. Cool down for 5 minutes.

12.4. Dinner: Carolina-Style Oven-Barbecued Chicken

Yield: 6 Servings

Ingredients

For Chicken:

1 teaspoon sugar

1 teaspoon garlic powder

1 teaspoon paprika

1/2 teaspoon ground allspice

1/2 teaspoon black pepper

1/4 teaspoon salt

1/4 teaspoon dry mustard

1/8 teaspoon ground red pepper

2 1/2 pounds skinless chicken thighs

For Sauce:

2 tablespoons vinegar

2 tablespoons water

1 tablespoon honey

1 teaspoon Worcestershire sauce

1/2 teaspoon (about) hot pepper sauce

1/2 teaspoon prepared mustard

6 hamburger buns, split, toasted

Instructions

Preparing the Chicken:

1. Pre-heat the oven to 375 F.
2. Mix the first 9 ingredients in a mixing bowl.
3. Massage the spice mixture onto the chicken thighs.
4. Position the chicken on a rack in a roasting pan.
5. Bake in the oven uncovered until the chicken is tender and no longer pink, approximately 45 minutes.
6. Allow the chicken to cool slightly.
7. Take the meat from the bones and shred.

Preparing the Sauce:

1. Mix the vinegar, water, honey, Worcestershire sauce, hot pepper sauce and prepared mustard in mid-sized saucepan.
2. Add in the shredded chicken and heat.
3. Apply the mixture onto hamburger buns.
4. Serve.

12.5. Dessert: Gingersnap Pumpkin Cheesecake

Yield: 12 Slices

<u>Ingredients</u>

Crust:

8 ounces gluten free gingersnap cookies

3 tablespoons butter, earth balance

Filling:

16 ounces cream cheese, dairy free (room temperature)

1/4 cup dairy free sour cream

1 (15 ounce) cans pumpkin puree

3/4 cup unrefined sugar

1 teaspoon vanilla

1 teaspoon ground cinnamon

1/2 teaspoon ground ginger

1/2 teaspoon ground cloves

1/2 teaspoon ground nutmeg

1 teaspoon cinnamon

1/4 teaspoon salt

2 1/2 tablespoons cornstarch

3 eggs, room temperature beaten

<u>Instructions</u>

1. Pre-heat oven to 325 F

Prepare Crust:

1. Apply a butter slightly along the sides of spring-form pan.
2. Melt the remaining butter.
3. Grind the gingersnap cookies in food processor then add the melted butter.
4. Apply by press mixture into pan.
5. Bake in the oven for 15-20 min until slightly brown.

Prepare Filling:

1. Boil water for water bath.
2. Blend cream cheese until smooth.
3. Add in sugar, sour cream, pumpkin, add beaten eggs, vanilla, spices and cornstarch and blend well.
4. Pour into crust.
5. Whenever the crust has cooled wrap the pan with foil then fill the baking pan with boiling water to half the height of the spring-form contents.
6. Place the cake into water bath.
7. Bake approximately for 1 hr. until the outside is set but inside is still a bit loose.
8. Turn oven off and leave door slightly open and leave cake in oven for another 30 minutes.
9. Cool on rack.
10. Slide a knife around the edges and refrigerate for 6-8 hours or overnight until firm.

Day 11

13.1. Breakfast: Dairy-Free Scrambled Eggs

Yield: 1 Serving

Ingredients

2 to 3 Large Eggs

Water

Dairy-Free margarine

Splash Unsweetened Milk Alternative

Kosher Salt, to taste

Freshly Ground Black Pepper, to taste

Instructions

1. Whisk the eggs with a few tablespoons of water.
2. Warm up some dairy-free dairy- free margarine in a skillet and then cook the eggs on low heat.
3. Carefully fold the eggs into the center of the pan.
4. Whenever the eggs are almost fully cooked, add a bit of the unsweetened milk alternative to the top of the eggs then turn off.
5. Apply with salt and pepper as preferred.

13.2. Lunch: Greek Salad

Yield: 6 Servings

<u>Ingredients</u>

1/2 cup extra-virgin olive oil

1 1/2 cup fresh basil kosher salt and black pepper

2 14-ounce cans stuffed grape leaves

8 ounces Non-Dairy Vegan Feta Cheese, broken into large pieces

1 seedless cucumber, peeled and cut into 1/4-inch half-moons

1 cup cherry or grape tomatoes, halved

1 12-ounce jar pepperoncini, drained

1 lemon, cut into wedges

3/4 cup olives, preferably kalamata

<u>Instructions</u>

1. In a blender, mix the olive oil, 1 cup of the basil, and ¼ teaspoon salt and place aside.
2. Separate the stuffed grape leaves, vegan feta, cucumber, tomatoes, pepperoncini, lemon, olives, and the remaining ½ cup of basil among plates.
3. Apply to the tomatoes and cucumber ¼ teaspoon each salt and pepper.
4. Drizzle over with the basil oil.
5. Serve.

13.3. Snack: Caramel Apple Cookies

Yield: 36 Servings

<u>Ingredients</u>

1/2 cup plus 2 tablespoons unsalted butter, softened

1 cup plus 2 tablespoons packed brown sugar

1 large egg

2 tablespoons non-dairy milk

3/4 teaspoon vanilla extract

6.75 ounces gluten-free flour (about 1 1/2 cups)

3/4 teaspoon baking soda

1/4 teaspoon salt

1 1/2 cups gluten-free old-fashioned rolled oats

2 chopped peeled apples

20 caramel candies

2 tablespoons water

<u>Instructions</u>

1. Pre-heat oven to 325 F.
2. Blend the butter and brown sugar with a mixer at mid-speed until creamy.
3. Add in the egg, non-dairy milk, and vanilla.
4. Mix for approximately 2 minutes or until light and fluffy.
5. Mix flour, baking soda, and salt in a bowl.

6. While stirring add in oats.

7. Add the oat mixture to butter mixture, beating at low speed then stir in apples.

8. Position dough by 1 1/2 tablespoonful's 2 inches apart onto baking sheets lined with parchment paper.

9. Bake in oven at 325 F for 14 minutes or until golden.

10. Transfer cookies to wire rack.

11. Cool down to room temperature.

12. Add caramels and water in a small pan.

13. Prepare over low heat 7 minutes, stirring till smooth.

14. Take away from heat.

15. Drizzle with warm glaze over cookies.

16. Allow to stand for 15 minutes or until caramel is completely set.

17. Serve.

13.4. Dinner: Super Quick Cheeseless Pizza

Yield: 4-6 Servings

<u>Ingredients</u>

Pizza crusts (gluten-free, or dairy-free)

Tomato sauce

Sliced or diced black olives

Fresh or dried oregano, optional

Crushed red pepper, optional

Uncured Salame

<u>Instructions</u>

1. Pre-bake pizza crust as instructed on packaging.
2. Top the pizza with sauce, followed by olives, oregano, crushed red pepper, and sliced salame.
3. Apply by overlapping as they will shrink slightly upon cooking.
4. Bake in the oven for 5 to 7 minutes, or until the crust is golden and the salame begins to sizzle.
5. If preferred, broil for a couple of minutes to crisp up the salame.

13.5. Dessert: Orange Delight Cake

Yield: 10 Servings

Ingredients

2 cups cake flour

1 1/3 cups white sugar

2 teaspoons baking powder

1/4 teaspoon baking soda

3/4 teaspoon salt

2 teaspoons orange zest

2/3 cup shortening

1/3 cup orange juice

1/3 cup water

2 eggs

2 tablespoons lemon juice

2 egg whites

1 1/2 cups white sugar

5 tablespoons water

1/8 teaspoon salt

1 1/2 teaspoons light corn syrup

1/8 teaspoon cream of tartar

1 teaspoon vanilla extract

2 tablespoons grated orange zest

1/2 cup chopped walnuts

Instructions

1. Pre-heat oven to 375 F.
2. Slightly grease and flour two 8 inch cake pans.
3. Combine together into a bowl the cake flour, 1 1/3 cups sugar, baking powder, baking soda, and 3/4 teaspoons salt.
4. Include grated orange rind, shortening, orange juice, and 1/3 cup water.
5. Blend on mid-speed for 2 minutes with an electric mixer, scraping bowl while blending.
6. Add in two whole eggs and beat batter for 2 additional minutes.
7. Add in the lemon juice then pour batter into the prepared pans.
8. Bake in the oven at 375 F for 30 to 40 minutes.
9. Take out the cakes from pans and allow to cool.
10. Frost with whipped cream if preferred.
11. Drizzle cake with grated orange rind and chopped nuts or coconut.
12. Serve.

Day 12

14.1. Breakfast: Baked Cinnamon Toast

Yield: 4 Servings

<u>Ingredients</u>

8 slices crusty bread, at least 1 inch/2.5 cm thick

8 eggs

3 cups rice or soy milk

3/4 cup pure maple syrup

1/2 tsp cinnamon

1/2 tsp nutmeg

Icing sugar (optional)

<u>Instructions</u>

1. Pre-heat oven to 350F.
2. Grease a 9 x 13 inch baking dish.
3. Position the bread snugly into the baking dish including more bread if required.
4. Slightly beat the eggs, then stir in the rice or soy milk, maple syrup, cinnamon, and nutmeg.
5. Apply the mixture over the bread.
6. Bake uncovered in the oven for 55-60 minutes or until golden brown and the middle is set.
7. Drizzle with icing sugar or additional maple syrup as preferred.
8. Serve.

14.2. Lunch: Horseradish Roast Beef and Vegan Cheddar Cheese Roll-Ups

Yield: 4 Servings

Ingredients

4 ounces non-dairy cream cheese, softened

2 tablespoons prepared horseradish

4 large flour tortillas

1 head romaine lettuce, tough remove the rib

8 ounces thinly sliced deli roast beef 4 ounces

Vegan Cheddar cheese, thinly sliced

Instructions

1. In a bowl, blend the non-dairy cream cheese and horseradish.
2. Distribute evenly over each tortilla.
3. Layer the tortillas with the lettuce, roast beef, and Cheddar.
4. Roll up tightly.
5. Serve.

14.3. Snack: Peanut Butter-Banana Spirals

Yield: 6 Servings

Ingredients

1/2 cup reduced-fat peanut butter

1/3 cup vanilla non-dairy yogurt

1 tablespoon orange juice

2 ripe bananas, sliced

4 (8-inch) fat-free flour tortillas

2 tablespoons honey-crunch wheat germ

1/4 teaspoon ground cinnamon

Instructions

1. Mix the peanut butter and non-dairy yogurt till smooth.
2. Drizzle the orange juice over bananas and toss.
3. Apply 3 tablespoons peanut butter mixture over each tortilla, leaving a 1/2-inch on the border.
4. Arrange 1/3 cup banana slices in a single layer over the peanut butter mix.
5. Intermix the wheat germ and cinnamon then sprinkle evenly over the banana slices.
6. Roll up tightly.
7. Slice each roll into 6 pieces.

14.4. Dinner: Watermelon Baja Fish Tacos

Yield: 12-16 Tacos

Ingredients

Watermelon Guacamole:

2 medium avocados, peeled and chopped
Chopped cilantro
1 can (4 ounces) diced green chilies, drained
2 tablespoons lime juice
2 teaspoons diced jalapeno pepper (or to taste)
2 medium garlic cloves, minced
1½ cups diced watermelon
Salt, to taste

Baja Fish Tacos:

Cooking spray
1½ pounds cod
Chili powder, to taste
Salt, to taste
12–16 corn tortillas
3–4 cups commercial coleslaw mix (shredded cabbage and carrots)
½–1 cup commercial salsa
1 cup diced watermelon

Instructions

1. Prepare the guacamole by mashing the avocados in a bowl until a mixture of smooth and chunky.
2. Place in the cilantro, green chilies, lime, jalapeno, and garlic and mix.
3. Include 1½ cups diced watermelon and salt and toss.
4. Cover up.
5. Heat oven to 350 F and grease a baking sheet.
6. Position the cod on sheet and sprinkle with chili powder and salt.
7. Bake for approximately 12–20 minutes.
8. Cut the cod into bite-sized chunks
9. Warm the tortillas on grill or griddle.
10. Add in each with few pieces of fish, ¼ cup coleslaw mix, heaping spoonful of guacamole, tablespoon of salsa and few of the leftover diced watermelon.

14.5. Dessert: Almond Cookies

Yield: 9 Servings

Ingredients

1 egg white, room temperature

1/3 cup coconut sugar

1/2 teaspoon almond extract

1/2 cup almond flour

1 tablespoon slivered almonds, chopped

Instructions

1. Pre-heat oven to 300 F.
2. Line an 8x8-inch baking dish with parchment paper.
3. Mix the egg white, coconut sugar, and almond extract.
4. Fold almond flour into egg mixture till well combined.
5. Add batter into baking dish.
6. Drizzle almonds over top of batter then press down slightly.
7. Bake in a pre-heated oven until golden brown, approximately 25 minutes.
8. Move cookies over to a cooling rack using the parchment to lift it out of baking dish.
9. Cool down to room temperature.

Day 13

15.1. Breakfast: Gingerbread Pancakes

Yield: 6-8 Servings

Ingredients

Vegan egg:

1 tablespoon ground flaxseed

3 tablespoons water

Dry ingredients:

1 cup whole wheat flour

1 serving vanilla plant-based protein powder

1 teaspoon baking powder

1/2 teaspoon baking soda

1 teaspoon ground cinnamon

1/2 teaspoon ground ginger

1/4 teaspoon freshly grated nutmeg

1/8 teaspoon ground cloves

Wet ingredients:

1 teaspoon apple cider vinegar

1 1/2 cups vanilla soy milk

1 tablespoon canola oil

1/2 teaspoon vanilla

1 tablespoon real maple syrup

Instructions

1. Prepare the vegan egg by stirring the flax meal and water in a bowl then place aside to thicken.
2. Intermix all the dry ingredients in a mid-sized bowl.
3. In another bowl, mix the apple cider vinegar and soy milk to create vegan buttermilk.
4. Include in and mix in the canola oil, vanilla, and maple syrup.
5. Add the flax egg.
6. Include the wet ingredients to the bowl of dry, and combines until mixed (try to avoid over mixing to prevent from looking gummy).
7. Prepare a pan over mid-heat and allow to warm up for approximately five minutes before cooking the pancakes.
8. Apply cooking spray, then pour about two tablespoons of batter onto the pan for each pancake.
9. When you see bubbles start to form, flip.
10. Cook for an additional minute.
11. Serve.

15.2. Lunch: Swiss Mushroom and Almond Melt

Yield: 4 Servings

Ingredients

4 slices whole-grain bread, lightly toasted

1 avocado, sliced

1 cup sliced mushrooms

1/3 cup sliced toasted almonds

1 tomato, sliced

4 slices Vegan Swiss cheese

Instructions

1. Pre-heat the oven broiler.
2. Position the toasted bread out on a baking sheet.
3. Add to each slice of bread 1/4 of the avocado, mushrooms, almonds, and tomato slices.
4. Add on top the slice of Swiss cheese.
5. Broil the sandwiches open until the cheese melts for approximately 2 minutes.
6. Cool and serve warm.

15.3. Snack: Tomato Turnovers

Yield: 12 Servings

Ingredients

8 (14 x 9-inch) sheets frozen phyllo dough, thawed

1/4 cup olive oil, divided

1 teaspoon freshly ground black pepper

1 cup multicolored grape tomatoes, quartered lengthwise

1/4 cup thinly sliced shallots

2 tablespoons chopped fresh basil

1 teaspoon chopped fresh thyme

1/4 teaspoon kosher salt

Cooking spray

Instructions

1. Pre-heat oven to 375F.

2. Position 1 phyllo sheet on a flat work surface (cover remaining phyllo to prevent drying) then lightly brush phyllo sheet with oil.

3. Add 1 teaspoon pepper evenly over phyllo then top with an additional phyllo sheet.

4. Add tomatoes, thinly sliced shallots, chopped fresh basil, chopped fresh thyme, kosher salt, and grate together in a bowl.

5. Arrange approximately 1/3 cup tomato mixture along short side of phyllo.

6. Roll up phyllo starting with the short side.

7. Slightly brush outside of roll with oil then cut into thirds.

8. Position on a baking sheet coated with cooking spray.

9. Repeat the procedure with remaining 6 phyllo sheets, pepper mixture, oil, and tomato mixture.

10. Bake in oven at 375 F for 10 minutes or until phyllo is golden.

11. Serve up warm or at room temperature.

15.4. Dinner: Oriental Beef with Broccoli

Yield: 1-2 Servings

Ingredients

1 pound flank steak, partially frozen

1/2 cup oyster sauce

1/4 cup water

3 tablespoons mirin or cooking sherry

1 tablespoon arrowroot powder or cornstarch

1/4 teaspoon crushed red pepper flakes

4 tablespoons peanut oil, divided use

1 tablespoon grated gingerroot or ¼ teaspoon ground ginger

1 clove garlic, minced

3 cups broccoli flowerets

1 red bell pepper, seeded julienned

1/2 cup diagonally sliced green onions

Instructions

1. Slice the partially frozen flank steak across the grain to make very thin 2×1-inch strips.
2. In a bowl, combine oyster sauce, water, mirin and arrowroot powder then stir until powder is well dissolved.
3. Add in crushed red pepper flakes and place aside.
4. Warm a large non-stick skillet or wok over mid-high temperature.

5. Include half of the peanut oil and heat until very hot
6. Add in the beef and stir-fry until browned, approximately 2 minutes.
7. Take away the beef from wok with a slotted spoon and place aside.
8. Warm the same skillet or wok over mid-high temperature.
9. Include the remaining peanut oil and stir-fry ginger and garlic for 30 seconds.
10. Add in the broccoli and stir-fry for 3 minutes.
11. Increase heat to high and add in red bell pepper and green onion then continue to stir-fry for another 3 minutes. Decrease heat to medium.
12. Place in beef and reserved oyster sauce.
13. Mix constantly until mixture thickens for approximately 1-2 minutes.
14. Serve up over brown or white rice.

15.5. Dessert: Dairy-Free Brownies

Yield: 8 Servings

Ingredients

1 cup vegan semi-sweet chocolate chips

1/4 cup canola oil

2 eggs, beaten

2 teaspoons instant coffee granules

1/2 cup white sugar

1/3 cup cocoa powder

1/3 cup gluten-free flour

1/8 teaspoon baking soda

1 tablespoon coffee-flavored liqueur

1 teaspoon vanilla extract

Instructions

1. Pre-heat oven to 350 F.
2. Heat up the chocolate with canola oil in a glass bowl in a microwave for 30 second increments, stirring until completely melted for 2 to 3 minutes.
3. Add in the eggs and coffee granules into the melted chocolate.
4. Mix sugar, cocoa powder, flour, and baking soda together into another bowl then add to the chocolate mixture and stir to combine.

5. Add in the coffee liqueur and vanilla extract into the mixture and stir.
6. Pour in the brownie batter into an 8-inch square baking dish.
7. Bake in a pre-heated oven until beginning to dry along the edges for approximately 20 to 25 minutes.
8. Cool down and serve.

Day 14

16.1. Breakfast: Quinoa Breakfast Bowl

Yield: 1 Serving

Ingredients

1/2 to 1 cup plain cooked quinoa

1/4 to 1/2 cup vanilla non-dairy milk (almond or hemp milk)

1 teaspoon liquid sweetener agave or maple syrup (if not using sweetened almond or hemp milk)

Cinnamon, nutmeg, and/or cardamom

Fresh fruit of your choice (about 1/2 cup)

A sprinkling of nuts and/or seeds

Instructions

1. Warm up the cooked quinoa in a small pan with a bit of non-dairy milk.
2. When most of the non-dairy milk has been absorbed, transfer over to a bowl.
3. Add in sweetener and spice as preferred.
4. Top with fruit, followed by nuts and seeds.
5. Serve up at once.

16.2. Lunch: Chipotle-Lime Grilled Fish Tacos

Yield: 6 Servings

<u>Ingredients</u>

Marinade:

1/4 cup extra virgin olive oil

2 tablespoons distilled white vinegar

2 tablespoons fresh lime juice

2 teaspoons lime zest

1 1/2 teaspoons honey

2 cloves garlic, minced

1/2 teaspoon cumin

1/2 teaspoon chili powder

1 teaspoon seafood seasoning, such as Old Bay™

1/2 teaspoon ground black pepper

1 teaspoon hot pepper sauce, or to taste

1 pound tilapia fillets, cut into chunks

Dressing:

1 (8 ounce) container dairy-free sour cream

1/2 cup adobo sauce from chipotle

Peppers

2 tablespoons fresh lime juice

2 teaspoons lime zest

1/4 teaspoon cumin

1/4 teaspoon chili powder

1/2 teaspoon seafood seasoning, such as Old Bay™

Salt and pepper to taste

Toppings:

1 (10 ounce) package tortillas

3 ripe tomatoes, seeded and diced

1 bunch cilantro, chopped

1 small head cabbage, cored and shredded

2 limes, cut in wedges

Instructions

Prepare the Marinade:

1. Mix together the olive oil, vinegar, lime juice, lime zest, honey, garlic, cumin, chili powder, seafood seasoning, black pepper, and hot sauce in a bowl.
2. Put the tilapia in a dish, and pour the marinade over the fish then cover and refrigerate 6 to 8 hours.
3. Prepare the Dressing:
4. Mix the sour cream and adobo sauce.
5. Add in the lime juice, lime zest, cumin, chili powder, seafood seasoning.
6. Include salt and pepper.

Prepare the Fish for Grilling:

1. Pre-heat the grill for high heat and lightly oil grate.
2. Position the grate 4 inches from the heat.

3. Take the fish from the marinade and drain off any excess.
4. Grill the fish pieces for approximately 9 minutes.
5. Put together tacos by placing fish pieces in the middle of tortillas with desired amounts of tomatoes, cilantro, and cabbage.
6. Drizzle with dressing.
7. Serve up by rolling up tortillas and garnish with lime wedges.

16.3. Snack: Pumpkinseed Mix

Yield: 6 Servings

Ingredients

2 cups gluten-free crispy rice cereal squares (such as Rice Chex)

1/2 cup salted roasted whole pumpkinseeds

1/3 cup slivered almonds

1 tablespoon canola oil

2 teaspoons chili powder

2 teaspoons Worcestershire sauce {Check for Gluten}

2 teaspoons prepared mustard

1/2 teaspoon Spanish smoked paprika

1/4 teaspoon ground cumin

1/4 teaspoon ground red pepper

Cooking spray

1/4 teaspoon salt

Instructions

1. Preheat oven to 300 F.
2. Mix first 3 ingredients in a bowl.
3. Blend the oil and next 6 ingredients in a small bowl; drizzle over cereal mixture, tossing well to coat.
4. Line a large jelly-roll pan with foil; coat aluminum foil with cooking spray.
5. Position the cereal mixture on prepared pan.

6. Place in oven and bake at 300F for 10 minutes then stir.

7. Continue to bake an additional 7 minutes or just until mixture begins to turn brown.

8. Take away from oven; sprinkle with salt, and stir.

9. Cool down in pan.

16.4. Dinner: Savory Salmon Burgers

Yield: 12 Burgers

<u>Ingredients</u>

1 pound salmon, skin removed

1 tablespoon toasted sesame oil

1 tablespoon ume plum vinegar

1 clove garlic, pressed

1 teaspoon peeled and minced fresh ginger

¼ cup chopped scallions (white and green parts)

¼ cup toasted sesame seeds

2 large eggs

1 tablespoon coconut flour

Coconut oil, for frying

<u>Instructions</u>

1. Rinse clean the salmon, pat dry and cut into ¼-inch cubes.
2. In a bowl, combine salmon, oil, ume, garlic, ginger, scallions, sesame seeds and eggs
3. Mix the coconut flour into mixture.
4. Make use of ¼ cup measuring cup to form mixture into patties.
5. Heat the coconut oil in a 9 inch skillet over mid-high heat.
6. Prepare the patties for 4 to 6 minutes per side or till golden brown.

7. Transfer patties over to a paper towel-line plate and serve up hot.

16.5. Dessert: Easy Lemon Bars

Yield: 16 bars

<u>Ingredients</u>

Crust:
1½ cups Almond Flour

5 tablespoons Tapioca Starch

¼ teaspoon Real Salt

2 tablespoons Honey

3½ tablespoons Butter, cold, cut into cubes

Topping:
4 Eggs

3 Egg Yolks

½ cup Honey

½ Cup + 1 tablespoon Fresh Lemon Juice

¼ teaspoon Salt

4 tablespoon Butter, cut into small cubes

3 tablespoon Coconut Milk (canned)

<u>Instructions</u>

1. Pre-heat the oven to 350 F.
2. Line a '9x9" baking pan with parchment paper.
3. In the bowl of the food processor, mix together the almond flour, tapioca starch, and salt.

4. Include the honey and cubes of butter and process until dough forms smooth.
5. Start to press the dough evenly into a 9x9" baking pan lined with parchment paper.
6. Place the crust in the oven for 10 minutes or just until it starts to turn golden brown on top.
7. To make the filling whisk together the eggs, honey, lemon juice, and salt until very smooth.
8. Set the pan on mid-high temperature and add in the butter cubes.
9. Blend constantly until the butter melts and the mixture starts to boil.
10. When the mixture boils, take away it from the heat.
11. Mix in the coconut milk and add the filling on top of the par-baked crust.
12. Place back in the oven and bake for an additional 10 minutes, or until the filling is glossy and set.
13. Allow to cool completely.
14. Place in the refrigerator for a couple of hours and slice into bars with a warmed knife.

Meet the Author

Diana Welkins' motivation is to encourage other individuals to embrace more plant-based healthy foods in their eating habits without feeling deprived in addition to an avid supporter of the occasional indulgence. She shares delectable, stimulating recipes that she takes pleasure in on a daily basis. Diana Welkins wants to encourage you to step into the kitchen to prepare a delightful, healthy and balanced meal.

Next Steps

-Write an honest review about the book – I truly value your opinion and thoughts and I will incorporate them into my next book, which is already underway.

Author's Page http://www.amazon.com/Diana-Welkins/e/B00WS76QHY/ref=ntt_dp_epwbk_0

Additional Recipe Books

Dairy-Free

Envious Cow Non-Dairy Ice Cream: 31 Flavors of Dairy-Free, Paleo, and Vegan Friendly Ice Cream Recipes

Dairy-Free Smoothies: Seriously Yummy Paleo, Vegan, and Gluten-Free Non-Dairy Smoothie

Slice The Dairy: 21 Tasty and Delicious Dairy-Free Pizza Recipes

Vegetarian

Vegetarian Cookout: Scrumptious Barbecue Grilling Recipe Cookbook

Vegetarian Freezer Meal Recipes: Time Saving Vegetarian Freezer Meal Recipes

Vegetarian Lifestyle Cookbook: 20 Delightful Vegetarian Lasagna Recipes

Paleo

30 Days Paleo Diet Breakfast: Ultimate Ready Paleo Diet Breakfast Meal Recipe Cookbook

No Grain, No Gain Sandwich Recipes: Premium Gluten-Free and Paleo Breadless Sandwiches and Wraps Recipes

Sneak Peek

Diary-Free Smoothies
Seriously Yummy Paleo, Vegan and Gluten-Free Non-Dairy Smoothies
By Diana Welkins

Are you currently searching for delicious and dairy-free smoothies designed to suit any diet?

Smoothies are a fantastic solution to sneak nutrition into any diet plan. Consuming hefty servings of fruit provides you with all the nutrients you will need in a simple and satisfying way! The perfect types of smoothies are non-dairy. All natural fruit smoothies provide you with more energy and are fulfilling, therefore smoothies are an easy way to start off your day. The fruits all-natural flavors will take control of the taste! If you would like a selection of terrific tasting and stimulating smoothie recipes, select Dairy-Free Smoothies.

Why are Diary-Free Smoothies the best option?

There are numerous explanations why non-dairy is the best option. Avoiding milk, ice cream and yogurt reduces lots of calories from your smoothie, and can actually be more nutritious. Regardless of whether it's a hot summer day or you are simply out of milk or ice cream. Consuming a dairy-free fruit smoothie will taste amazing, and make you feel rejuvenated. Similar to almost all smoothies, these are fairly inexpensive and simple to make, so let us get to mixing!

Equipment You Will Need to Make a Great Smoothie

Before you start, you will need a very good blender. You will need a blender that can tear up and blend food of all textures quickly. There are many varieties of fruits you will be using. It is essential to have a blender that can quickly and effectively crush ice, so a good quality blender is preferred. I'm sure you have a blender already, but it could be time for an upgrade. You can search through Amazon for a good quality blender.

To read more visit [Dairy-Free Smoothies: Seriously Yummy Paleo, Vegan, and Gluten-Free Non-Dairy Smoothie](#)

Made in the USA
Coppell, TX
04 October 2023